Healthy Breast After Cancer and Treatment

Healthy Breast After Cancer and Treatment

My Story

Valerie R. Morris

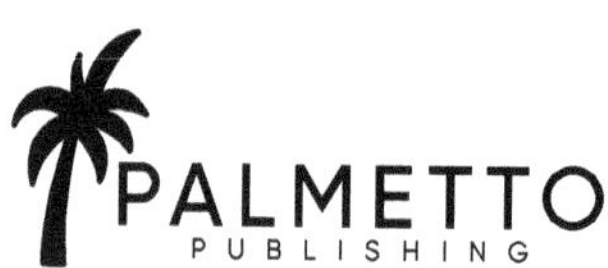

Charleston, SC
www.PalmettoPublishing.com

Healthy Breast After Cancer and Treatment

Paperback ISBN: 978-1-64990-935-0

Table of Contents

Introduction

MY STORY

My adventure started at the end of January 2007.I was going to my annual visit to the Gynecologist, she said "everything looks good you just need to have your mammogram done". I went to the appointment had the pictures taken and left.

I was called back for additional pictures as the previous ones were not clear. I arrived for the appointment and this time the radiologist was available to read the films before I leave. They proceeded to do an ultrasound, took pictures and said my doctor would call with the results. Now during the test, the technician will not tell you anything, I tried. You will have to wait for your doctor to call and tell you whatever news the technicians and radiologist found.

My gynecologist Dr. L. R. called to say that they did find a spot on my left breast and that would need to be biopsied. "Okay", my mind is going crazy with this information. First thing I think of is cancer, I really did not want cancer of any kind. My sister C passed last April with complications (Tongue cancer, Lung cancer & Crohn's, she was 11 months younger than me). I am the oldest of the 3 girls, so the sooner I had this checked out, the better I would feel.

I could not wait so I made some phone calls to places that did breast biopsies. I found a place and called my doctor to let her know what I found, but she did not know the other doctor in question and asked if I would wait one day? I said I would wait.

My Dr. L. R. called to say she scheduled an appointment for the next day for me to see a breast surgeon who would do a biopsy of the spot on the left breast. It was the Breast Health Center at Women& Infants Hospital. I met with Dr. J.G. who explained that my mammogram showed a spot on the left breast, and that she would need a biopsy on that area to see if it is cancer or something else. I agreed because my maternal grandmother's sister (great aunt) had breast cancer in her 90's, she had a mastectomy back then.

Now first and foremost you need to like the doctors you have working for you because you will be seeing them for the next 5 years. This is very important.

I had the biopsy right there in her office. She proceeded to numb my left breast with Lidocaine, she took out a large needle; this is what she calls a Needle Aspiration. Let me tell you I do not like needles of any kind and this one is big, it scares me, I know big baby, yup. I close my eyes and stay very still so she can take multiple samples and then she stops. She patches me up sends me home with an appointment for the following week.

I went back for the results hoping that it was good news, but it turned out that yes it was cancer. Dr. J.G. makes an appointment with radiology to do a biopsy of the left arm pit lymph nodes with dye.But radiology found 2 more locations that need to be checked and biopsied. I go to this appointment and they prep me for the ultrasound, they need to find the spots from the mammogram and then call the doctor in to numb me and to do a biopsy on them. The technician cannot find the spots she just found. They schedule and MRI of both breast and biopsy of the left with a dye contrast for the following week.

The technicians prep me for the MRI. They numb my left breast then they place me in the machine and look for the spots. They find the spot and proceed to clamp down my left breast to make sure I do not move while the doctor takes the samples. My surgery is in 2 weeks.

To tell you the truth I am scared shitless, but I am waiting for confirmation before I say anything. It is easier that way.

Now I must tell my mom that I do have breast cancer and the 20 other females, who are cousin's, niece's and my own baby sister R who is 6 years younger. They need to know the possibility of them getting it. My family and friends are supportive which is helpful. My husband was there through the whole thing.

The day before surgery I go to Diagnostic to be injected with the dye to highlight the sentinel Node so that the doctor can take it out and further test it for cancer. Dr. J.G. believes the cancer is Ductal Carcinoma in situ stage 2, which means localized cluster of cancer cells in the milk ducts but have not penetrated the surrounding tissues. The MRI confirmed that there are 2 more spots, she will see to these during surgery.

Due to some allergies it was a learning experience for my doctor. The intern working with Dr. G proceeded to go on-line to make sure there was no problems during surgery. Thank god there was none.Surgery went well, it is a new type of surgery used. Cryosurgery was the type I had. This is where the area in question with additional parameters added, frozen and then removed. An example: using an egg that is boiled you then remove the yolk which would be the cancer and extra. I was told what and what not to do and be back for my next appointment, then I was sent home. I was a little sore but overall fine.

A week later I was told that I had stage 1 not 2 and the size was 1.4cm not 2.2cm, the lymph nodes had no cancer. This was good news, but I still need to get the radiation done.

Because I was given a heavy dose of antibiotics I ended up with a fungal infection in my mouth.Thrush hurts when you swallow; it can be anything, water or food. Food hurts more, so the following appointment I was given a prescription to clear that up.My next appointment after that was to meet the new Oncologist. My oncologist was a man, that is ok but as the appointment continues, I find I do not like this man.He may specialize in cancer, but I do not know, it just does not feel right. So when scheduling my next appointment. the girls ask how things are and I told her I just could not warm up to him. The girl said do not worry we will schedule you with another doctor every week until we find the right one. I did find one, Dr. R. S.

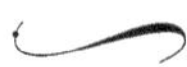

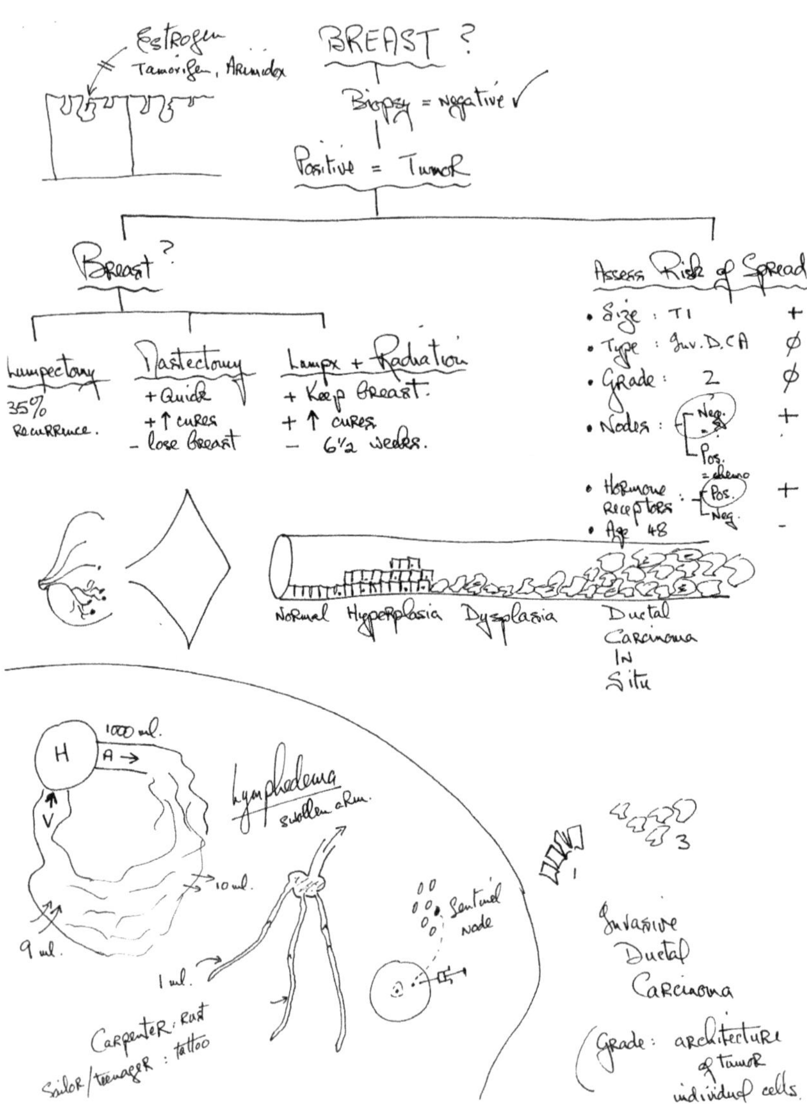
Estrogen
Tamoxifen, Arimidex
BREAST ?
Biopsy = negative
Positive = Tumor
Breast ?
Lumpectomy
35%
Recurrence.
Mastectomy
+ Quick
+ ↑ cures
- lose Breast
Lumpx + Radiation
+ Keep Breast.
+ ↑ cures
- 6½ weeks.
Assess Risk of Spread
• Size : T1 +
• Type : Inv. D. CA ϕ
• Grade : 2 ϕ
• Nodes : Neg. Pos. +
= chemo
• Hormone Receptors : Pos. Neg. +
• Age 48 -
Normal
Hyperplasia
Dysplasia
Ductal Carcinoma In Situ
H
A →
V
1000 ml.
10 ml.
9 ml.
1 ml.
Lymphedema
swollen arm.
Sentinel node
Carpenter : Rust
Sailor/teenager : tattoo
1
3
Invasive Ductal Carcinoma
Grade : architecture of tumor
individual cells.

I called up the Maddox Radiology for my radiation treatments. The doctor explained about my cancer. He said the type of cancer was "Ductal Carcinoma ", it did not penetrate the milk duct walls. A picture was even drawn so I knew what he was explaining. But he would ask about the type of treatment I was receiving. I said the lumpectomy and radiation. He then asked if I was having chemotherapy. He then said for treatment that the chemotherapy therapy needs to be first then radiation. I did not know this. I was told after surgery I needed a doctor in oncology, I did that. Now I needed to find out why someone told him I was doing chemotherapy. I tried to reach my new oncologist who it seems was not available all day. I called back the next day and spoke to the one I did not warm up to. He explained that the decision was up to me. Well I was getting angry and said "I still did not understand why I was not getting a clear answer to my question". I finally asked what my options were. I had a 10 – 15% chance of it coming back, I could opt for chemotherapy or forgo it altogether. By now I was angrier for the simple fact that I had been telling all the doctors I did not want the chemotherapy.

If they (the doctors) had been a lot clearer with the information on this, my decision would be Radiation and it would have already been started sooner than later. Once I told them my decision was no chemotherapy I called Dr. M and set up the schedule for radiation treatments. Radiation takes 6 ½ weeks or 32 days along with medication for 5 years call" Tamoxifen".

The first visit was in May, Dr. M tells me he is going to tattoo my left breast and when he finishes, he then sends me down the road for a Cat Scan.

He wants to make sure they are in the right spot. I also met the doctor helping with the radiation, Dr. B who informs you what you can use on your skin during radiation and she checks your skin to make sure the radiation is not burning it. I tried telling her that I personally cannot used Dove moisturizing soap, I break out in hives. But this is the soap they require you to use. I personally cannot use it.

I go to my visits and one day Dr. B said your skin looks great, the Dove works well. I said I am using Dial, she just looked at me and I told her I could only use Dial orange which she said was the harsh one. But I do not break out in hives, so I am still using it.

On one of my visits with the breast surgeon I was asked if I wanted to do the Taylor trial, but the cost is$1000. TAILORx Trials is short for Trial Assigning Individualized Options for Treatment(RX).This is used for women with early stage breast cancer. Now that is a lot of money, so I said I would see if I could raise the money.But it was short lived because that test needs to be done before your surgery to get an accurate test reading. The cancer cells must range 1.0mm and mine was .5mm, I was not a candidate so that ended that. Life goes on.

I started working again, I am a landscape gardener. The job is interesting and it is also physical, so because of my job the surgeon and oncologist recommended the Lymphedema clinic. Because they removed some lymph nodes, they wanted to make sure that my arm would not swell due to the loss of said lymph nodes. I went once a week and gradually progress to once a month. Going to the clinic was not only beneficial it was also therapeutic.Just think when you go to your appointment you get something called a soft body massage, very relaxing. I went at the end of my workday. I also continued helping my stepfather with my mother who has severe COPD. In all this time my mother was more worried about me than herself. All my appointments and that was seeing the surgeon, the oncologist, the radiologist, and my regular appointments were kept. I may have missed a day or two of work, but over all I went to all of them.

During all this time I have spent time with my mom. Whether it was after work or on days off I would be at her house. She is getting worse and now she is worried about her great grandson who is living in foster care in Northern RI, 30 minutes away. One day she said,"Valerie could you become a foster parent and have Andrew move in with you until his mother gets her act together," oh mom I do not know? That is so much more work and with everything else that is going on. But what my mother wanted she usually got. We would do just about anything for her. I became a foster parent at 49. Talk about starting over with my youngest at 24. Oh boy.I enrolled him in our schools I took him to the doctors to make sure he was healthy.

I am still working but my days are cut short because I needed to be at day care by a certain time. My son helps with Andrew with homework along with my husband. It has changed some since I went to school. And now we have a routine to follow.

I was approaching my 1st year anniversary I was counting the days. But by the end of January my mom took a turn for the worst. Arrangements were made for my niece to get Andrew back for February 1st of 2008; my mom passed February 2 of 2008. Her fight had ended, I followed her wishes and let her go to be with her parents and my sister C. It was the hardest thing for my stepfather and I could do, to stop the oxygen that was keeping her alive. My brothers, stepbrothers, sister and step-sister and spouses were there and said goodbye. She was gone. There was no funeral, she was cremated and will be buried with my stepfather when it is his time.

My 1st year anniversary came and went with no re-occurrence of the cancer. My life continued with mammograms every 6 months and seeing the surgeon and the oncologist.I continued visiting with my stepfather every day after work to make sure he was taking care of himself. When I was not working,I would take him to his doctor appointments or just spend time with him. He missed my mom so when his son and wife took their family on a cruise and offered to take him; I told him he needed to go and to at least enjoy being with his son and family. He came back with some color from being in the sun and he seemed more like himself before mom. He would tell my sister R and I that we were his girls and not to forget it, along with his own daughter, his first girl. We would be happy every time I had to go for mammograms, and they would be clean.

In March 2009, I was driving with my stepdad when a woman in a jeep broad sided my car, not once but twice. She said she missed the brake. I was able to get out of the car, but the passenger front door was bashed in. My stepdad was not sure if he was ok and I would not let him move as he had heart surgery years before, but I was not taking any chances. He ended up being alright.

This accident I hurt my right shoulder. I was told I have a bone degenerative disease, I ended up with a Rotor Cup Tear.

While out of work I was helping my cousin R. E. who was having health issues. Because of my breast cancer she was getting checked by my doctors. I do not know the results for her tests, but it was something to do about her health insurance. I ended up taking her to her OBGYN doctor who said he would remove the problem. The next thing I know he is cutting her boob with no lidocaine nothing. He was cutting out her milk ducts. When she screamed he told her to shut up and to stop screaming, my hand was sore from her squeezing it. I told her I was not going to take her to that quack. Her husband took her after that. In the end R. E. had breast cancer.

I continued to work and go to doctor appointment. My right shoulder started bothering me since the car accident so I had it check and I am told that my rotor cup is bad and I need surgery. I cannot have surgery now it will have to wait until the winter, in the meantime I am sent to therapy so that I can strengthen the muscles before I have surgery.Well I continue working and doing what was needed to be done and waited to schedule surgery.

But at the end of October 2009, while having my annual mammogram something was on the films. I was scheduled for an Ultrasound Biopsy, I was given lidocaine and just like the first time they find it and then they can't when their ready with the Needle Aspiration to take the samples. They find an opening for the MRI, clamp me in, find the spots and take the samples but by this time the lidocaine is wearing off. I bite hard clamp my jaw and get the rest of the test done. I can finally go home after about 3 hours.

I was told the day before mom's birthday that the cancer had come back in the same breast.This time it is called "Ductal Carcinoma in situ stage 2". This is because it has come back a second time.My first surgery was done Cryo-genetically meaning it was frozen and then removed. Unfortunately for me they missed one little cell who was hiding and now 2 ½ years later I have the same thing again.

So, on December 8, 2009 I had a double mastectomy, I did not want a re-occurrence in the right breast. I am also having a reaction to the tape holding the bandages to my chest. The skin is blistering, I am told to use Neosporin, this made it worse. Paper tape worked the best, no reaction. I am allergic to latex, which sometimes are on our bandages.

I would have had my reconstruction done the same day as my mastectomy but the Plastic Surgeon who was doing the surgery was going on vacation, so I had to wait. Also due to my job I would need to schedule it in the winter during my off season. I would have the winter off to recover and start work in the spring. The doctor also changed my medication from Tamoxifen to Arimedex for another 5 years.

I do my exercises from Dr J. G. my breast surgeon. I need to start raising my arms so that they will be straight up in the air. I am doing very well, and she is impressed with my range. I continue seeing my other doctor and I need to schedule surgery for a procedure from my gynecologist, Dr S. S. I feel like I am going in for repairs, like your cars.

It is now 2010 and I have scheduled February 3rd, with Dr. S.S. and I also need to schedule for Rotor cup surgery with Dr T.

B. which is February 21st. This is a hum dinger of a month. With all these surgeries I feel like a pin cushion but with all this done I hope for a smooth recovery so I can go back to work.

It is warming up so that I can work, I am being careful, but I hate slowing down.The fresh air does a body good for it is exhilarating to get out and work. I am enjoying work, to get out doors and work the soil and clean up winters mess it is exhilarating. To see daffodils, tulips popping their heads out of the ground. Then the azalea's, cherry and maple trees start to come in bloom, it is just so pretty. But because I cannot use my right hand correctly because of the shoulder surgery, I have created pain in my left wrist and thumb. What else will pop up from this mess I am in. But that does not stop me from doing some work.

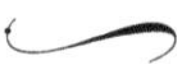

Now I must see some other doctors for this problem. The hand specialist diagnosed me with a trigger thumb and stress on the left wrist from using it incorrectly and the treatment was silly putty and cortisone shots. I was happy that they had a fix for my hand but when they gave the cortisone shots, one in the thumb and the other in the wrist, they really hurt. But it did help, and I was slowly retaining strength in my hand and my shoulder. It is the end of my season, so, on to step 2.

I have scheduled my first Reconstruction surgery for December 2, 2010 I wake up in ICU with my doctor asking how I am doing? My eyes popped out of my head when all I saw was my boobs in my face. Granted there are a lot of bandages, I looked at him and said, "what happened? I did not want to be this big", he told me it was just swollen from the surgery. Do not worry it will go down. I stayed in the hospital for a couple days so that they could keep an eye on me and to show me how to maintain the drain hoses that were in my chest. I was to document how much fluid was in each plastic container connected to the drain tubes, and what color is the fluid.I was sent home and told to come back for the next visit at his Dr. P.M's office.

Now that I am home my stepfather comes to my house to check on me instead of the other way around. It makes him feel useful when he is with me I am finally getting all the drains removed after having them for a couple weeks. It feels like freedom, no more tugging, or swinging when you do not catch it in time. But I ask my plastic surgeon again "about how long does it take for the swelling to go down? My chest is way too large. I was a B cup and now I am a triple D. I want to be smaller. He said again that "the swelling will go down it just takes time".

In the meantime, I am completely overwhelmed with everything that must be done with my treatment. The doctor just repeated himself with the swelling and I have to start chemo soon. Because the cancer came back I have to have chemotherapy. You cannot have Radiation twice.

I talk to Dr. J.O my primary doctor about everything that is going on and he said "you need to talk to someone who is not family or friend, you need to just release everything that's going on".

It was a good call as now my stepfather is having a bad cough that will not go away, so I take him to my pulmonologist to find out why he cannot stop coughing. A CT scan is ordered but I was not in the meeting for the results, he told me there was nothing they could find.

I need to go back to work, I just cannot deal with all the things that are going on and that are out of my control. So, I go back to a counselor that I have seen in the past when things get to be too much. I go for my visit and she ask how I been. I told her " I have had better days"; and I need her to help me focus and to organize my thoughts and how to proceed with my life, family and my health. I fill Dr. K.J my counselor in on all the things that have been going on. I told her that with everything that "I believed no one would miss me other than my stepfather and husband and a couple of friends". That I did everything I was told to do to make sure the surgeries done to my body would make a difference. That in my opinion was false because the reconstruction did not go like he explain. That I am a triple D and not a B. That I should not worry because of the swollenness, it takes time. This is May 2011 and my surgery was December 2, 2010; how long does it take? I was even going to the lymphedema clinic to help with any swelling that arises.

I continue working I am getting my range of motion back which makes my job easier.I start sneezing and coughing, ok probably someone mowing the lawns; I am allergic to fresh cut grass. But oh my god I get a pain in the area of both hips that drop me to my knees.Wow, what just happened? That really hurt and I do not know why.

This pain continues and every doctor that I go to has no idea what it is. They have appointments for me to see doctors in psychiatry, neurology, ultrasounds, acupuncturist and I also go and see Dr. R. C a chiropractor.

I am still having issues with my right shoulder. It is not better I think it is worse. I go to the shoulder surgeon who did the surgery he said that the surgery did not work that he could give me a cortisone shot and because of his future move I could continue with him as my doctor, but I would need to go to Conn. *I said "Yes, to the cortisone and no" to Conn." I went to my chiropractor, I love my Chiropractor, Dr R.C* he gave me the phone number to an orthopedic surgeon who worked on shoulders and he was located near me.

My shoulder hurts so bad that I am waking up at night with so much pain in my shoulder that I have to sleep sitting up. This is not comfortable. And it has been to long since surgery.

I still go to my appointment to see my counselor Dr. K. J she asked how I am doing today, And I think about it and tell her everything just does not seem to get better. Yes, my health and cancer seem to be better and gone but my stepfather is getting worse. Cough suppressants with codeine are not helping and his doctor even tried plain honey on a spoon to coat the throat.

Nothing seemed to work. Because I cannot do anything about it I have to let it go; for now.

I make an appointment to see this orthopedic surgeon for my shoulder, he is young so that's good, I guess. I just want this pain to all go away. I have pain in my right shoulder, pain in my chest and sharp pain in both hip areas. I know I can be a pain in the butt, but no one deserves to go through this. So, for everyone who goes through this I say I know how you feel and maybe with all this research maybe the younger ladies will not have to deal with all this crap. If I had only the breast cancer to deal with, the problems might not be this aggravating and painful, but I will never know that answer. With multiple surgeries it was done and there is nothing that can be done to change it, it's the past but hopefully we all can learn from this.

I was so busy with work and doctor appointments that I do not remember where or what I was doing. But my brother, CP calls me and ask why I had our stepfather intubated? I really had no idea what he was talking about? He told me he was at the hospital and that he was in ICU with our stepfather who has a tube down his throat. I told him " I was on my way". I get there and request seeing the doctor. When Dr. L.P came, he told me that " my stepfather was having a hard time breathing and he was not getting better. That it was time". I absolutely could not believe what was happening. I made phone calls to brothers, stepbrothers, stepsister and my sister, and CP help with the calls and requested that they come to RI right away because their dad was on life support and that there will be a meeting with his doctor when they got there.

All his children and stepchildren were there, and we all agreed to let him go and took him of life support, it was May 20th., It was a terrible time because this was when we all found out that he was living on credit and he was swamp in debt.

After all siblings sat at the dining room table all 9 of us really saw how bad it was. Their home he lived in had exceeded the value to over $80,000. He carried over 20 credit cards, there was no money left from mom's life insurance. Now my stepdad could do no more for the people who were leaching off of him, their sugar daddy had passed on. I need to find a lawyer who can help me as I am the executor of his will.

So, I asked all my siblings if there was anything that they wanted? Just let me know and they wrote it down on a pad of paper. My brothers, CP & F helped catalog everything in the house plus pictures were taken for proof of the items. It was 30 years of collecting everything they liked. I wanted to work to avoid the stress but then I would have to leave to go to a doctor's appointment that would be an hour away; this cut into my free time and work time.

I had to tell the rest of my family that I was in charge and that according to probate court I needed to lock up the garage as there was materials and tools inside it. I had my niece T.M and her husband call the police on me because they refused to stay out of the garage that I keep locking back up. The police told them to get their things out of the garage and then proceeded to arrest T.M 's husband on an outstanding warrant, R.M stayed in jail over the Columbus Day weekend.

The police stayed for a few minutes to make sure that we were keeping the peace. Now when my niece emptied the garage of their things, she took everything. Even tools and materials belonging to her grandmother, grandfather and uncles. It was completely empty and there was nothing I could do to prove that, so I let it go. After that they continued to play havoc with the tenants (stepdad rented out a duplex), and the property.I wanted this to go to probate, and that way we could close this part.

But the free time was not always fun. During the probate of my parent's estate, my niece T.M and my nephew J.M did not want to accommodate me or what I needed to do for probate. I would get phone calls from my brothers, CP & F telling me someone broke into the house. I had to call the police to report it, the break in, and what was missing. Then have to get the town water department to turn the water off at the main, because someone cut out all the copper pipes in the basement of the little cottage, but no one saw anything.

Well life in February 2011, I will have a procedure done by my gynecologist, just under 3 weeks later, which was no fun. I was

going to get my shoulder fixed. But because I had cancer on my left side you cannot use that arm for blood work or IV's. But I was having surgery on my right shoulder. Where were they putting the IV? I found out the day of surgery when the nurse who does the IV tells me it has to be put in the top of my foot. Let me tell you I screamed for that sucker hurt like hell. I hope I never have to go through that again.

Now I need to visit the plastic surgeon who will be doing the reconstruction (2nd surgery), but I need to heal from the 2 surgeries that was just done.

I am back at work, spring has arrived, but I am limited with my shoulder. At times like this I tell myself, that life really sucks. But I have a group of friends who have been with me during this whole mess. They all tell me to jus.t take my time, that the job will get done either way.

My primary doctor sends me to a pain management doctor who ask why I was sent to him?I told him about my surgery and that if I sneeze, cough or hiccup I drop to my knees in pain and could he help, I would appreciate it.

Well,he told me he was going to give me a nerve block and he hoped it worked. Dr. E. K solved my problem, I had no pain I was in heaven. Thank You. It is August 4; it has been 7 months and something finally works.

But it was short lived because the pain came back the following day. Well back to square one. I continue seeing doctors to determine what is causing this pain.

I am going to my counselor biweekly. Some days are better than others. I am still working and going to every doctor thrown at me, the pain in my hips are so bad I feel like a hypochondriac and I am not one.

I have an Acupuncture appointment to see if this type of medicine will help. I am not thrilled to be here as I have said before I hate needles, and this doctor is going to stick some in me. Yuck! Well it seems to help in some areas but the pain is still there. I come back a few times, but I would like to go to someone closer to my home.

At the end of October my oncologist sends me for a Gall Bladder ultrasound to see if this is from the pain I am having. But no, that is not it either, my gall bladder is fine. They all tell me I am healthy and I look well but they cannot determine why there is pain in my hips. So, I am continuing the acupuncture and the lymphedema clinic and I will eventually find out what has happened to me.

I have scheduled a second reconstruction surgery by Dr. P.M this is to down size my triple D chest to a B cup. I will also have exploratory surgery in the hips to find out why I have pain. I have met a general surgeon who will be there to see if she can find out why there is pain in the hip area. After the surgery I ask if this Dr. C.D the general surgeon, found anything related to this hip pain? Dr. P.M said she was not needed so no they do not know why there is pain. Talk about a patient's rights to have someone else in their surgery. Well because this pain was not getting better I continued seeing doctors.I feel like no one will figure this out.

After 81 visits to doctors and specialist this doctor look at my history, ask some questions and gave his diagnosis. When I had my first reconstruction, they did a tummy tuck. They slice you from "hip to hip", this is where I was having my pain; a general surgeon finally found out why I was in pain and it was because the nerves were sliced and were eventually growing back which was causing the pain.

After seeing Dr. M.J, I called my primary Dr. J.O who had me call Dr. E.K and schedule the nerve blocks. In March, I had 2 nerve blocks on each hip, 5 cm from my belly button. What a weird feeling when it's done. It's like having balloons expanding where they inject the medication. What a difference a nerve block can do. After a couple days of discomfort, I had no pain from my hips. I found out the first injection Dr. E.K did was only temporary.

I still did therapy for my shoulder and life was getting better. I work in client's yards and I enjoy it because there were no issues with my body. My 2012 work season was the best for I had finally found the best way to challenge and conquer the problems I had. I still have pain in my boobs and left ribs but it is becoming the normal.

December 2012, I had Dr. F.M take care of my right shoulder. Cortisone shots helped when I needed it but now to fix it. The first surgery in early 2011, did not correct the problem. What he found was an anchor and sutures from that surgery. When Dr. F.M finished he repaired the Rotor cup and three Labral tears that were away from the bone.

I am looking for another plastic surgeon, the one I have does not listen when I explain the pain I was having and still have in the boobs and left rib. So far none of the doctors I have seen cannot help due to the type of surgery, a TRAM (Transverse Retus Abdominis Myocutaneous) I had done. Found out later John Hopkins Hospital stop this type of surgery due to the side effects, which are risks of hernia's or abdominal bulge. I have the abdominal bulge along with pain in both breast (which is my own body fat). I am not sure if the other cancer patients have this problem, but I cannot put any pressure on the bulge area without excruciating pain. I cannot use my body to open jars or lean against some structure to get things. It is very frustrating.

In September 2013, I saw another plastic surgeon Dr. R.Z. First, I got lost going to his office and then fell face first on the side walk, going into his office. It did not turn out well from there. I explained that I needed smaller breast and would hope he could help. This man did not like having a fellow surgeon's work ridiculed. It did not matter that the patient was not happy. When I finally left, I was a basket case.

When I requested the consult notes, his 2 pages went down to 1 page. Wonder what else he called me. I also called my doctor's and insurance company about his bed side manner. I have never recommended him as a surgeon and I never will.

My family lost R.E., her fight has ended. She he is no longer in 1) pain and 2) or worried about how others feel. She is with the rest of the family, enjoying life.

October 2013, I fell in my dining room onto both of my knees. I had Dr. F.M my Orthopedic surgeon who had a MRI taken. My right knee needs work. Yippee. I just do not have it in me to have another surgery. I was given a cortisone shot and this is working for now.

2014 I had no real issues with my body on all the surgeries, but I still get pain in both breasts and in the left ribs. I am still trying to solve this problem. But one thing at a time.

2015; I went to a Lymphedema therapist L.D to see if she could help. L.D measured my arms and ordered the sleeves for both arms. I am still looking for a plastic surgeon and I have an appointment with Dr. W.R, he is older and I hope he will help. He has reviewed my history and Dr. W.R explains that a lot of doctors do not take on cases like this because they do not know what the other surgeon has done. But if I call the first surgeon and have them talk to each other he will do the next surgery on me. I have seen the doctor a couple times now and will be scheduling this surgery, it is called Reconstruction & Reduction of pre-existing TRAM.

March 2015, Dr. F.M proceeded to repair my right knee, radiology said the tear was on one side and Dr. F.M said it was the other side. I said "Look at both sides, ok, which ended up being double meniscus tear. When I started work it was the best because my knee did not bother me anymore. Life is good again, just wish there was an answer to breast and rib pain. But over all in all the years that past this is the last problem.

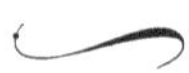

It is December 2015 and Dr. W.R. is scheduled to do this surgery for January 4,2016.My Reconstruction/Reduction of pre-existing TRAM.

January 4,2016

I wake up in recovery and I feel a difference in my chest. It is so much lighter; I am thrilled that I am so much smaller. The doctor said that the reduction came out well and we will see about the rest after I have healed some. I have order new lymphedema sleeves this year to help with any swelling. But there still is pain in the breast and ribs.

To be able to work more easily now, not banging into the boobs. I can wear regular clothes.I have a small group of Dr.s now that I still go to but over all it is a lot less visits.

I go back to Dr. W.R. in April 2017 to be re - evaluate, it is still bulgy under my breast. Is there any way to flatten this area out? Well, he said loose a little more weight and then he would be able to liposuction the excess fat from my first surgery and then tighten up under the breast with a fine seam to close it. Alright, but is there any way to reverse the abs back where they were? Dr. W.R said he would see if there is any way to do that but thought, no it cannot be done. In the meantime, I am losing weight and will see what happens.

March 2018 one of my toe's had an ingrown nail, went to a Podiatrist who took care of the problem but said"are your feet always cold? I said yes". I made the appointment to have the test done. I am having Circulation test done to all extremities. Did not think anything about it. Well the test involved pressure cups on both arms and legs. I know, left arm, no pressure readings, bloodwork or surgeries. I was lucky, my arm was tender for a couple days and then fine, but it could have been so much worse. I am still complaining about the breast pain and rib pain. I am having a CT Scan and Chest x-rays. I have signed up with the hospitals PORT to review my medical history and there it was. The results from the chest x-ray was three clips on my left ribs, exactly where my pain is.I have talk to my doctor and asked if the clips can be removed? The answer is no, so as of now I do not know if I can have this corrected or live with it.

That was May of 2019 and so far, there are no solution, but I plan on continuing this until it can be resolved. I am still working with my surgeon to see if he can correct this type of surgery, only time will tell. It is the end of the year and I go to my Dr.s once a year now. Gives me more time to do other things.

It is November 2020, I have lost about 20 pounds and plan to loose more. But with a pandemic going on in the world I will wait until it is safe to go for the last surgery. I am still trying to solve the clips on my ribs but have not found anything on it yet. But every day is a little better than the last. Only time will tell if I beat this and get my body back, then everything will be good in the world.

I have also been trying to figure out how the cancer started, yes there is my families genes but there was two more women who had breast cancer at the same time as me. If it was from my family then what about the other women, they are not related to me. So where did it come from; I live near a site that remove they say solvents, degreasers, PCP's, and contaminated fuel oil. Can that give you cancer? I do not know that answer, but it is strange all 3 women had some type of breast cancer at the same time. So far we are all alive and that is the plus we need.

I hope my story helps some one other woman to see a better picture of what goes on after surgery, thank you for listening.

Valerie

Chapter 1

ALL FEMALES WHO ARE SEXUALLY ACTIVE SHOULD START VISITING A GYNECOLOGIST.

Reason:

You are going to be checked annually for abnormalities; like cervical, ovarian or uterus cancer. There are also venereal diseases that can be transmitted between partners.

Establishing a relationship with your gynecologist is beneficial to your health, they ask many questions about you once they review your family history.

We as individuals let them use this information so they're able to determine what is important for health. That along with the annual exam, with a regular doctor.

Regular testing:

Blood work ......annually

- *CBC (white blood count)*
- *Cholesterol, Gastrointestinal*
- *Kidney Disease*
- *Heart Disease Cancers*

Pap Smear -annually

- *Abnormalities in cell formation in the cervices*
- *Venereal disease and cancer*

Mammogram's begin at the age of 40, higher risks the age is 30

This is to view the interior of the breast, to see any lumps, cyst or cancer spots.

Results from the mammogram...can be normal or there could be shadows. Picture is not clear due to fatty mass in the breast. Additional pictures or an Ultra - Sound is performed.

Ultra- sound shows something. The next step is to have an Ultra - sound biopsy. Still not enough information to diagnose you will need an MRI.

Magnetic Resonance Imaging or MRI......will detect 91% of cancers.

MRI with Contrast is when a dye is injected into the arm to high light area needing to be viewed.

MRI Biopsy is when samples of the breast tissue are taken for testing.

Magnetic Breast Imaging (MBI) ...dye is injected into arm to high light area to get a camera shot to a mammogram.

Chapter 2

CANCER IS DIAGNOSED

First Stage

- *Determine next how bad is bad*

- *Lumpectomy: removal of cancer and the sentinel and other lymph nodes*

- *Surgery is done; your next step is Radiation Therapy, and cancer medication for next 5 years*

- *Depending on the severity of the cancer you may need to have chemotherapy also, this is determined by your surgeon.*

Second Stage

- *Cancer is reoccurring*
- *Mastectomy and removal of more lymph nodes*
- *Chemotherapy and medication for next 5 years.*
- *Information found Family Circle "NO RETURNS"Adjuvant chemotherapy.Single Boost of Radiation Treatment with Aromatase inhibitors Femara Gene Base Testing*

Lymph node Removal

- *Lymphedema Clinics should be started as soon as your doctor lets you.Reason is that with the removal of your lymph nodes you have a higher risk of getting lymph-edema. This is where your arm swells up because the lymph nodes are gone. They help the body sweat which releases excess fluid.*

Chapter 3

STAGES

0 TO IV

Stage 0 is non-invasive or no evidence of cancer

Stage 1 is when cancer cells are breaking through or invading clean breast tissue with tumors up to 2 cm and none of the lymph nodes are attacked

Stage 2 has 2 categories

1. *IIA is invasive but no tumor is found but cancer is found in the lymph nodes or the tumor measures 2 cm or smaller and spreads to the axillary (under the arm) lymph nodes.*

2. IIB is invasive and the tumor measures 2 cm but not larger than 5 cm and has not spread to the axillary lymph nodes.

Stage 3 has three categories, IIIA, IIIB, IIIC.

1. IIIA is invasive but no tumor in the breast tissue, but cancer is found in the axillary lymph nodes.The cancer is clumping together or sticking to other structures or has spread to the lymph near the breastbone or cancer of any size spreading to axillary lymph nodes and clumping to other structures.

2. IIIB is invasive and the cancer is any size and has spread to the chest wall or the skin of the breast and may also spread to the axillary lymph nodes with clumping or sticks to structures and or spreads to the breastbone.

   Inflammatory Breast Cancer is considered stage IIIB because typically a larger portion of the breast tissue is red and swollen also warm to the touch. Cancer cells spread to the lymph nodes and maybe found on the skin.

3. IIIC is also invasive with no signs of cancer in the breast or the tumor is any size and spreads to the,chest wall. And or skin of the breast and the cancer has spread to the axillary lymph nodes or to the lymph's near the breastbone.

Stage IV is invasive and has spread beyond the breastbone and the nearby lymph nodes to other organs in the body.Example is the lungs, distant lymph nodes, skin, bones, liver or the brain. This stage represents advanced or metastasized. This happens first time or when cancer is reoccurring.

Chapter 4

TNM STAGE IS TUMOR, NODES, METASTASIS

Three (3) characteristics are

1. *Size (T is Tumor)*
2. *Lymph node involvement (N stands for Nodes)*
3. *Whether cancer has metastasized (M stands for Metastasis)*

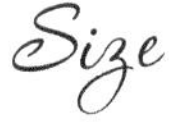

***TX** means there is no tumor to be measured*

***TO** means no evidence of a primary tumor*

T1 means cancer is In-Situ (tumor has not started growing in the healthy tissues of the breast)

T1, T2, T3, T4 are numbers based on the size of the tumor and to what extent that has compromised those healthy tissues.

N means your lymph nodes

NX means nearby lymph nodes can't be found or measured

NO means nearby lymph nodes have no cancer

N1< N2, N3,are based on the number of lymph nodes found with cancer, the higher the number the higher the amount of cancer.

M means metastasis and this means the cancer has traveled to other parts of the body.

MX means cancer can't be found

MO means no distant metastasis

M1 means distant metastasis is present

These are all the terms found on the pathologist report the doctor receives from the lab.

Example of a report: T1 NO MO will mean thatT1 has a primary tumor that is less than2 cm

NO *means there is cancer in the lymph nodes at the time of testing.*

MO *means that the cancer has not spread through the body.*

(all this information was found on the internet under www.breastcancer.org)

Chapter 5

LUMPECTOMY & LYMPH NODES

This is done surgically by removing the area in question also the removal of some of your lymph nodes that are under your arm, they will be sent to the lab for further testing.

RADIATION

This procedure is done by a specialist in Radiology who will pinpoint the area that needs to be radiated, treatment will vary from 33 days or more.

CHEMOTHERAPY

This is done intravenously in the arm (on the opposite side of where the cancer was found) with a special cocktail (specific drugs combination) that will kill the cancer cells in question. Depending on the severity of the cancer will depend on how many treatments needed to kill all the cancer cells.

REOCCURRING

When treating cancer for the first time, most patients will go through radiation and not do the chemotherapy, especially if the cancer's ratio of coming back is small. If the cancer comes back it is reoccurring and the only option is chemotherapy.

MASTECTOMY & LYMPH NODES

If the cancer is severe on the first diagnoses your doctor could recommend that a mastectomy is your only option. If it is reoccurring your option will be a singular or bilateral mastectomy. This is where they will remove one or both breast and to also so remove lymph nodes under your arm.

These samples are sent the laboratory for testing.

Chapter 6

LYMPHEDEMA CLINIC

With the removal of your axillary lymph nodes (under your arm) your doctor will recommend you go to the clinic. This will ensure that your arms are treated so that there will be no swelling. When loosing the lymph nodes our body has the tendency to swell due to buildup of fluids. Our body's natural sweating system is no longer working properly. The clinic has therapist who are trained to massage the arm to train it to release fluids differently. I look at it as the therapist are building new roads to release excess water. This can take a couple of months or longer.

Chapter 7

MAMMOGRAMS

What age to start

For women who are not a high risk the age starts at 40 years old, every 2 years are recommended.Now, high risk individuals, who has breast cancer in their family is age30. Mammogram are used to detect any abnormalities in the breast tissue.To check the area they will do an ultra -sound to determine what is there, this will give a better picture.If something is there you will be scheduled with a surgeon. A needle biopsy is a more accurate test.If nothing is there your mammogram will be done twice a year

Mammograms and Others

What age to start

Regular mammograms start at the age of 40.

For females with a higher risk, should have mammograms done at age 30.

REGULAR MAMMOGRAMS

Mammograms are done once a year, usually when you have a yearly exam with your gynecologist

ABNORMAL MAMMOGRAMS

When your mammogram is abnormal you will need to follow up with your Doctor and have a mammogram done twice a year.

ADDITIONAL PICTURES

This can be done either by more mammograms, ultra -sound or MRI (Magnetic Resonance Imaging)

ULTRA- SOUND

This procedure is done by applying a gel to the skin and scanning the skin surface to review on a computer screen where they take a picture of the area in question.

ULTRA -SOUND BIOPSY

Is the same procedure but then the breast is injected with a numbing agent, then the doctor comes in to inject a special needle that takes samples of your breast tissue.

MRI

It's magnetic resonance imaging and this is another test that gives a better pictures vs ultra -sound and the mammograms. For those with a higher risk with the heredity geneBRCA1 and BRCA2, you should consider having this done cost is about $2000.MRI's detect 91% of cancers.

MRI WITH CONTRAST

The doctor injects a radioactive agent into your arm, this allows the chemical to highlight the areas that the doctors are focus on.

MRI BIOPSY

This is done after the agent is injected, then the breast is clamped into place so that you don't move. The breast is numbed, then the special needle is used to take samples for testing.

Chapter 8

DIAGNOSED WITH CANCER

What Types of Cancer

Ductal Carcinoma

Forms in the lining of the milk ducts.

Ductal Carcinoma In-Situ (DCIS)

This means that it is inside the ductal system of the milk duct forms precancerous lesions

Lobular Carcinoma in-situ (LCIS)

Is not precancerous and non-invasive, will not evolve but increases risk in both breast.

Milk producing lobules- starts in the lobule of the breast where milk is produced.

Invasive- infiltrating outside the membrane ducts or lobular.

Connective tissues- begins in the connective tissue that make up the muscle, fat and blood vessels.This is called Sarcoma's

Infiltrating Ductal Carcinoma (IDC)

This is lesions that appear star like (stellate) or rounded (well circumscribed). there is about 78% of Malignancy

Medullary Carcinoma

Represents about 15% of cancers types that frequent women ages,late 40's & 50's cells resemble grey matter

Infiltrating Lobular Carcinoma (IBC)

This is when the breast tissue thickens in the upper outer quadrant of the breast,this cancer represents 5% of all diagnosis. It also responds to hormone therapy

Tubular Carcinoma

Makes up 2% of cancer diagnosis found in women ages 50 and over.

Mucinous Carcinoma (Colloid)

Makes up 1% - 2% of carcinomas. This is a mucus producing and the cells are poorly define.

Inflammatory Breast Cancer(IBC)

This one is rare and aggressive, causes the lymph vessels in the skin of the breast to be blocked. This cancer is called inflammatory because the breast itself looks red and swollen. 1% to 5% of all breast cancers cases are in this category.

Cancers Fueled by Hormones

ER - *Estrogen receptor positive -sensitive to estrogen*

PR - *Progesterone receptor positive - sensitive to progesterone*

Hormone block medication - *tamoxifen to slow cancer growth is used for ER & PR*

HR - *Hormone receptor negative - does not have receptors and does not respond to hormone based therapy.*

HER-2 gene - *is "human epiderma growth factor receptor2. Cancer cells that have many copies* *of HER – 2 gene. Medication is available to shut down growth of cancer. HER2 is not normally tested on Ductal Carcinoma in Situ.*

(this information was found on the web under (www.nationalbreastcancer.org)

Chapter 9

CANCER

Diagnosed with Cancer

First Stages

- *Lumpectomy & Removal of Lymph nodes*
- *Radiation*
- *Chemotherapy*

Second Stages

- *Reoccurring*
- *Mastectomy & Removal of Lymph nodes*

- *With the removal of lymph nodes there is the potential of getting Lymphedema.This is where your arms will swell up because the lymph nodes cannot work correctly because of the removal of lymph nodes.*

Lymphedema clinic

- *Go as soon as you can, I believe this is a necessary for overall health.*

Chapter 10

DEFINITELY CANCER

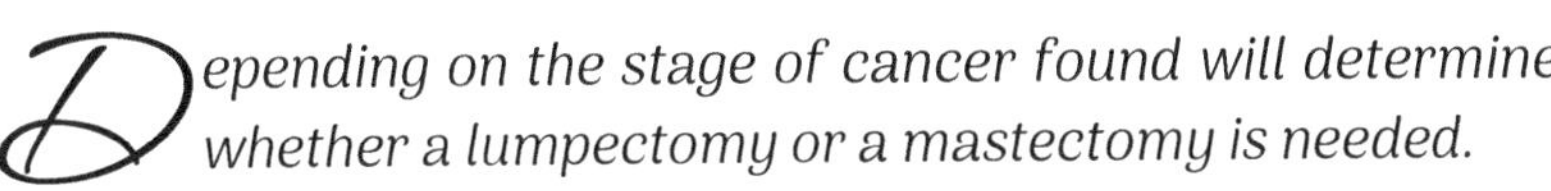

Depending on the stage of cancer found will determine whether a lumpectomy or a mastectomy is needed.

Lumpectomy

- *Go to the hospital for 1 – 3 days*
- *Cryosurgery is when they freeze the cancerous area, and then removing it.*
- *Dye is injected to locate the sentinel lymph node.*
- *Some lymph nodes are removed along with the sentinel for testing of cancer cells.*
- *Samples are taken around surrounding areas to ensure cancer free.*

- *Regular visits to the surgeon, radiation, oncologist etc. the list goes on, just to stay cancer free.*

Mastectomy

- *Depending on your type of cancer you have, is it the first time or the second time determines your procedure.*
- *You've had your biopsy done and now the decision is to remove your breast or both.*
- *All the testing has been done and now you go forward.*
- *Blood work is done*
- *Injected with the contrast dye to locate the sentinel lymph node to aid in the removal of additional lymph nodes, in the area of the cancer.*
- *Your given anesthesia and then wheeled into surgery.*

Chapter 11

AFTER SURGERY

Follow up visits to

- *Breast surgeon*
- *Radiation Treatments*

If cancer is severe

- *Chemotherapy*
- *Oncologist every 6 months*
- *Medication Taken for 5 years*
- *Tamoxifen & Arimidex are some*

www.ingramcontent.com/pod-product-compliance
Ingram Content Group UK Ltd.
Pitfield, Milton Keynes, MK11 3LW, UK
UKHW020421250726
13967UKWH00007B/2750

9 781649 909350